The Disease Fighting Meal:

How to Use Food to Prevent and Reverse Life-Threatening Illnesses

ROBERT R. THOMAS

TABLE OF CONTENT

INTRODUCTION

The Disease-Fighting Diet: How to Use Food to Prevent and Reverse Life-Threatening Illnesses

The power of food to heal and prevent disease is well-established in scientific literature. From heart disease to cancer, diabetes to Alzheimer's, research has shown that a healthy diet can prevent and even reverse many chronic illnesses. Despite this knowledge, many people continue to rely on medications to manage their health, overlooking the potential of a healthy diet to prevent and treat diseases.

The Disease-Fighting Diet is a comprehensive guide to using food as medicine. In this book, we will explore the latest research on how certain foods and nutrients can prevent and reverse life-threatening illnesses. We will provide practical tips on how to incorporate these foods into your diet and create healthy eating habits that will last a lifetime.

Part One of the book will cover the science behind food as medicine, including the role of nutrients, inflammation, and the gut microbiome in preventing and treating disease. Part Two will focus on specific diseases, such as heart disease, diabetes, and cancer, and provide evidence-based recommendations on how to use food to prevent and reverse these illnesses.

Part Three will provide practical tips on how to adopt a disease-fighting diet, including meal planning, grocery shopping, and cooking. We will also provide guidance on how to overcome common obstacles such as time constraints, budget limitations, and food preferences.

The Disease-Fighting Diet is not a quick-fix solution, but rather a long-term approach to health and well-being. By adopting a disease-fighting diet, you will not only prevent and reverse chronic illnesses, but also improve your energy, mood, and overall quality of life. The journey may not always be easy, but the rewards are immeasurable.

We hope that The Disease-Fighting Diet will inspire you to take control of your health and empower you with the knowledge and tools necessary to live a vibrant, disease-free life. Let's begin the journey to optimal health together.

PART ONE: THE SCIENCE OF DISEASE PREVENTION

CHAPTER 1

Food as Medicine – The Science Behind Disease Prevention

The old adage "You are what you eat" is more than just a saying. The food we consume has a direct impact on our health, and research has shown that a healthy diet can prevent and even reverse many chronic diseases. In this chapter, we will explore the science behind food as medicine and how it can prevent diseases.

Nutrients and their Role in disease prevention

Nutrients are essential for the growth, development, and maintenance of the body. They play a crucial role in preventing chronic diseases such as heart disease, diabetes, and cancer. Nutrients such as antioxidants, fiber, and healthy fats are found in abundance in whole foods, such as fruits, vegetables, whole grains, and nuts.

Inflammation and its Impact on Disease

Inflammation is the body's natural response to injury or infection, but chronic inflammation can lead to many diseases, including heart disease, diabetes, and cancer.

Inflammation in the body can be promoted or reduced by the food we eat. Foods high in sugar, refined carbohydrates, and unhealthy fats can promote inflammation, while whole foods such as fruits, vegetables, and healthy fats can reduce inflammation.

Gut microbiome and disease prevention

The gut microbiome is a collection of bacteria, fungi, and other microorganisms that reside in the gut. The gut microbiome plays a crucial role in maintaining our health by aiding digestion, regulating the immune system, and producing essential nutrients. The food we eat can either promote a healthy gut microbiome or disrupt it, leading to many diseases such as obesity, diabetes, and inflammatory bowel disease.

Plant-based meals

Plant-based meals are rich in fiber, antioxidants, and other nutrients that are essential for good health. They are also low in saturated fat and high in healthy fats, which can help reduce the risk of heart disease.

The impact of processed foods on disease

Processed foods are high in sugar, unhealthy fats, and refined carbohydrates. These foods have been linked to many chronic diseases, including heart disease, diabetes, and cancer. Processed foods also lack essential nutrients such as fiber and antioxidants, which are necessary for good health.

In conclusion, food can be a powerful tool in preventing and even reversing chronic diseases. Nutrients, inflammation, gut microbiome, plant-based diets, and processed foods all play a crucial role in the science behind food as medicine. Eating a diet rich in whole foods such as fruits, vegetables, whole grains, nuts, and healthy fats can promote good health and prevent many chronic diseases

CHAPTER 2

A Healthy Heart: Foods to Prevent and Reverse Heart Disease

Heart disease is the leading cause of death worldwide, and its prevalence continues to increase. However, research has shown that a healthy diet can help prevent and even reverse heart disease. In this chapter, we will explore the foods that can help you maintain a healthy heart and avoid heart disease.

Fruits and vegetables

Fruits and vegetables are rich in vitamins, minerals, fiber, and antioxidants, all of which are essential for a healthy heart. Studies have shown that people who consume more fruits and vegetables have a lower risk of developing heart disease. It is good to get at least 5 servings of vegetables and fruits daily.

Whole grains

Whole grains such as oats, brown rice, and whole wheat are rich in fiber, which can help lower cholesterol levels and reduce the risk of heart disease. Aim for at least 3 servings of whole grains per day.

Lean protein

Choose lean protein sources such as skinless chicken, fish, and legumes instead of red meat, which is high in saturated fat. Saturated fat can raise cholesterol levels and increase the risk of heart disease. Aim for 2-3 servings of lean protein per day.

Nuts and seeds

Nuts and seeds such as almonds, walnuts, and flaxseeds are rich in heart-healthy fats, fiber, and other nutrients that can help lower cholesterol levels and reduce the risk of heart disease. Aim for a handful of nuts or seeds per day.

Fish

Fatty fish such as salmon, tuna, and mackerel are rich in omega-3 fatty acids, which can help reduce inflammation and lower the risk of heart disease. Aim for at least 2 servings of fatty fish per week.

Olive oil

Olive oil is rich in monounsaturated and polyunsaturated fats, which can help lower cholesterol levels and reduce the risk of heart disease. Use olive oil instead of butter or other saturated fats when cooking.

Low-fat dairy

Low-fat dairy products such as skim milk and low-fat yogurt are rich in calcium and other nutrients that can help maintain a healthy heart. Choose low-fat dairy products instead of full-fat dairy products, which are high in saturated fat.

Dark chocolate

Dark chocolate contains flavonoids, which are antioxidants that can help lower blood pressure and improve blood flow to the heart. Aim for a small piece of dark chocolate per day.

Green tea

Green tea contains antioxidants that can help lower cholesterol levels and reduce the risk of heart disease. Aim for at least 2 cups of green tea per day.

In conclusion, a healthy diet is essential for a healthy heart. Incorporating these heart-healthy foods into your diet can help prevent and even reverse heart disease. Always go for a balanced diet that includes a variety of fruits and vegetables, whole grains, lean protein, nuts and seeds, fish, olive oil, low-fat dairy, dark chocolate, and green tea

CHAPTER 3

Breathing Easy: Foods to Prevent and Treat Lung Diseases

The health of our lungs is critical to our overall well-being. Unfortunately, due to environmental pollutants and lifestyle choices, many people suffer from lung diseases such as asthma, chronic obstructive pulmonary disease (COPD), and lung cancer. While medication and other therapies can help manage these conditions, diet can also play a significant role in both preventing and treating lung diseases.

Antioxidant-rich Foods: Antioxidants can help reduce inflammation in the lungs and protect against cellular damage caused by free radicals. Foods that are high in antioxidants include berries, dark leafy greens, nuts, and seeds.

Omega-3 Fatty Acids: Omega-3s are known for their anti-inflammatory properties and can help reduce inflammation in the lungs. Foods that are high in omega-3s include fatty fish, such as salmon and tuna, flaxseed, chia seeds, and walnuts.

Vitamin D: Studies have found that people with low levels of vitamin D are more likely to develop lung diseases. While vitamin D can be obtained from sunlight, foods such as fatty fish, egg yolks, and fortified dairy products can also be good sources.

Magnesium: Magnesium is essential for healthy lung function and can help reduce inflammation in the airways. Foods that are high in magnesium include dark leafy greens, nuts, seeds, and whole grains.

Garlic and Onions: These foods contain compounds that can help reduce inflammation in the lungs and improve immune function.

Turmeric: Turmeric contains a compound called curcumin, which has been shown to have anti-inflammatory and antioxidant properties. It can help reduce inflammation in the lungs and also improve respiratory function when it is added to the diet.

Ginger: Ginger has been used for centuries to treat respiratory conditions, including asthma and bronchitis. It contains compounds that can help relax the muscles in the airways and reduce inflammation.

Water: Staying hydrated is essential for healthy lung function. Drinking enough water can help thin mucus in the lungs, making it easier to cough up.

Avoiding Harmful Substances: In addition to eating a healthy diet, it is also important to avoid substances that can harm the lungs, such as tobacco smoke, air pollution, and secondhand smoke.

While diet alone cannot cure lung diseases, incorporating these foods into your diet can help improve lung function and reduce inflammation. If you suffer from a lung disease, be sure to talk to your healthcare provider about the role that diet can play in managing your condition.

Part II: Boosting Brain Health with Food

CHAPTER 4

The Mind Diet: Foods to Prevent Alzheimer's and Dementia

Alzheimer's and dementia are devastating conditions that can rob people of their memories, independence, and quality of life. While there is no cure for these diseases, recent research suggests that the right diet can help prevent or delay their onset.

In this chapter, we'll explore the latest science on the link between diet and cognitive health, as well as the specific foods that can help protect your brain from dementia and Alzheimer's disease.

The Mind Diet and Cognitive Health

The Mind Diet is a new eating plan that has been specifically designed to reduce the risk of Alzheimer's and dementia. The diet is a combination of two other popular eating plans: the Mediterranean diet and the DASH diet.

The Mediterranean diet is rich in fruits, vegetables, whole grains, nuts, and olive oil. It has been shown to reduce the risk of heart disease, stroke, and other chronic conditions. The DASH diet, on the other hand, is designed to lower blood pressure and is rich in fruits, vegetables, whole grains, and low-fat dairy products.

The Mind Diet combines the best of these two diets and has been shown to improve cognitive function and reduce the risk of Alzheimer's and dementia by up to 53%.

Foods That Protect Your Brain

So, what are the specific foods that can help protect your brain from cognitive decline?

Leafy Greens: Leafy greens are rich in vitamin K and have been shown to improve cognitive function and reduce the risk of dementia.

Berries: Berries like blueberries, strawberries, and raspberries are rich in antioxidants, which help protect the brain from oxidative stress and inflammation.

Whole Grains: Whole grains like oats, quinoa, and brown rice are high in fiber, which helps reduce inflammation and improve cognitive function.

Nuts: Nuts like almonds, walnuts, and cashews are high in healthy fats, which help protect the brain from cognitive decline.

Fish: Fatty fish like salmon, mackerel, and sardines are rich in omega-3 fatty acids, which have been shown to improve cognitive function and reduce the risk of Alzheimer's and dementia.

Beans: Beans like black beans, kidney beans, and chickpeas are high in folate, which has been shown to reduce the risk of cognitive decline.

Olive Oil: Olive oil is rich in monounsaturated fats, which help protect the brain from cognitive decline.

Wine: Red wine in moderation has been shown to have antioxidant properties and may help protect the brain from cognitive decline.

Incorporating these foods into your diet can help improve your cognitive function and reduce your risk of Alzheimer's and dementia.

Conclusion

While there is no cure for Alzheimer's and dementia, research suggests that a healthy diet can help prevent or delay their onset. The Mind Diet, which is a combination of the Mediterranean and DASH diets, has been specifically designed to protect the brain from cognitive decline.

Incorporating leafy greens, berries, whole grains, nuts, fish, beans, olive oil, and red wine into your diet can help improve your cognitive function and reduce your risk of Alzheimer's and dementia. By eating a healthy diet, you can help protect your brain and enjoy a higher quality of life as you age.

CHAPTER 5

Nourishing the Brain – Foods to Treat Cognitive Decline

Cognitive decline is a common issue among older adults, and it can significantly impact their quality of life. Memory loss, difficulty with problem-solving, and decreased attention span are some of the most common symptoms of cognitive decline. While there are many factors that contribute to cognitive decline, including genetics and lifestyle choices, recent research has suggested that certain foods can help prevent or even reverse cognitive decline.

The Importance of Nutrients for Brain Health

The brain is an incredibly complex organ that requires a variety of nutrients to function properly. Some of the most important nutrients for brain health include omega-3 fatty acids, B vitamins, vitamin D, and antioxidants. Omega-3 fatty acids, found in fish like salmon and mackerel, are important for brain function and can improve memory and cognitive performance. B vitamins, particularly vitamins B6, B9, and B12, are essential for brain function and can improve cognitive performance in older adults. Vitamin D, found in fatty fish and fortified foods, is important for brain health and can reduce the risk of cognitive decline. Antioxidants, found in fruits and vegetables, can protect brain cells from damage and reduce the risk of cognitive decline.

Foods for Brain Health

Several foods have been shown to be particularly beneficial for brain health. Berries, particularly blueberries, and strawberries, are rich in antioxidants and can improve cognitive function. Leafy greens, such as spinach and kale, are rich in nutrients and antioxidants that can protect brain cells and improve cognitive function. Whole grains, such as brown rice and quinoa, are rich in B vitamins and can improve cognitive performance in older adults. Fatty fish, such as salmon and mackerel, are rich in omega-3 fatty acids and can improve memory and cognitive performance.

The Role of Gut Health in Brain Health

Recent research has also suggested that gut health plays an important role in brain health. The gut microbiome, the collection of bacteria and other microorganisms that live in the gut, can impact brain function and cognitive performance. Probiotic-rich foods, such as yogurt and kefir, can improve gut health and promote cognitive function. Additionally, prebiotic-rich foods, such as bananas and onions, can promote the growth of beneficial bacteria in the gut.

The Benefits of Occassional Fasting for Brain Health

Occassional fasting is a pattern of eating that involves periods of fasting and periods of eating, has also been shown to be beneficial for brain health. Intermittent fasting can improve cognitive function and reduce the risk of cognitive decline by promoting the growth of new brain cells and reducing inflammation.

Conclusion

In conclusion, while the cognitive decline is a common issue among older adults, certain foods and lifestyle choices can help prevent or even reverse cognitive decline. A diet rich in omega-3 fatty acids, B vitamins, vitamin D, and antioxidants can improve brain function and reduce the risk of cognitive decline. Foods such as berries, leafy greens, whole grains, and fatty fish are particularly beneficial for brain health. Additionally, promoting gut health through probiotic- and prebiotic-rich foods and intermittent fasting can also improve brain function and reduce the risk of cognitive decline.

CHAPTER 6

The Gut-Brain Connection – How Food Affects Digestive Health

The digestive system is a complex network of organs and tissues that work together to break down food and absorb nutrients. While we often think of digestion as a purely physical process, recent research has shown that there is a strong connection between the gut and the brain. This connection, known as the gut-brain axis, is a complex network of communication pathways that allows the gut and the brain to communicate with each other.

The Role of the Gut Microbiome

The gut microbiome, the collection of bacteria and other microorganisms that live in the gut, plays a crucial role in the gut-brain axis. The gut microbiome helps to digest food, absorb nutrients, and regulate the immune system. It also produces neurotransmitters, such as serotonin and dopamine, that play a key role in regulating mood and cognitive function. The balance of bacteria in the gut microbiome can impact a wide range of bodily functions, including digestion, immune function, and mental health.

Foods for Digestive Health

The foods we eat can have a significant impact on the health of the gut microbiome and the gut-brain axis. A diet that is high in fiber, particularly from fruits, vegetables, and whole grains, can help to promote the growth of beneficial bacteria in the gut. Fermented foods, such as yogurt, kefir, and sauerkraut, are also rich in beneficial bacteria and can help to support a healthy gut microbiome. In contrast, a diet that is high in processed foods, sugar, and unhealthy fats can disrupt the balance of bacteria in the gut and contribute to digestive issues.

The Impact of Stress on Digestive Health

Stress can impact the gut-brain axis and digestive health. Chronic stress can lead to inflammation in the gut, which can disrupt the balance of bacteria and contribute to digestive issues. Additionally, stress has the tendency to impact the production of neurotransmitters, such as serotonin and dopamine, which can also impact mood and cognitive function.

Lifestyle Choices for Digestive Health

In addition to diet and stress, there are several lifestyle choices that can impact the gut-brain axis and digestive health. Exercise has been shown to promote the growth of beneficial bacteria in the gut and reduce inflammation. Getting enough sleep is also important for digestive health, as sleep helps to regulate the production of hormones that impact digestion and appetite.

Conclusion

In conclusion, the gut-brain axis is a complex network of communication pathways that plays a crucial role in digestive health. The gut microbiome, the collection of bacteria and other microorganisms that live in the gut, plays a key role in the gut-brain axis and can impact a wide range of bodily functions. A diet that is high in fiber and fermented foods can help to support a healthy gut microbiome, while stress and unhealthy lifestyle choices can disrupt the balance of bacteria in the gut and contribute to digestive issues. By making healthy food choices and practicing stress management and healthy lifestyle habits, we can support the health of the gut-brain axis and promote optimal digestive health.

CHAPTER 7

Colon Cancer Prevention – Foods to Keep Your Gut Healthy

Colon cancer is a serious health concern that affects millions of people worldwide. While there are many factors that can contribute to the development of colon cancer, including genetics and lifestyle choices, recent research has shown that diet plays a crucial role in colon cancer prevention. In this chapter, we will explore the foods that can help to keep your gut healthy and reduce your risk of colon cancer.

Fiber and Colon Health

Fiber is a crucial nutrient that plays a key role in digestive health. A diet that is high in fiber can help to keep the digestive system running smoothly and reduce the risk of colon cancer. Fiber promotes regular bowel movements and also helps to prevent the build up of waste in the colon that can result to cancer. Additionally, fiber helps to feed the beneficial bacteria in the gut microbiome, which can help to support overall gut health.

Foods for Colon Health

There are several foods that are particularly beneficial for colon health. Fruits and vegetables, particularly those that are high in fiber, such as broccoli, Brussels sprouts, and berries, are excellent choices for colon health. Whole grains, such as brown rice, quinoa, and whole wheat bread, are also rich in fiber and can help to promote digestive health.

certain nutrients have also been shown to be particularly beneficial for colon health. Calcium, for example, has been shown to reduce the risk of colon cancer. Foods that are high in calcium, such as dairy products, leafy greens, and fortified plant-based milk, can help to promote colon health. Vitamin D is another nutrient that has been shown to reduce the risk of colon cancer. Foods that are high in vitamin D, such as fatty fish, egg yolks, and fortified foods, can help to support colon health.

Unhealthy Foods and Colon Health

In contrast to the foods that promote colon health, there are several foods that can increase the risk of colon cancer. Processed meats, such as bacon, sausage, and deli meats, have been shown to increase the risk of colon cancer. Additionally, a diet that is high in red meat has been associated with an increased risk of colon cancer.

While it is not necessary to eliminate these foods from your diet entirely, it is important to limit your consumption of processed and red meats and to focus on a diet that is rich in fruits, vegetables, and whole grains.

Conclusion

In conclusion, diet plays a crucial role in colon cancer prevention. A diet that is high in fiber and nutrient-dense foods, such as fruits, vegetables, whole grains, dairy products, and fatty fish, can help to promote colon health and reduce the risk of colon cancer. In contrast, a diet that is high in processed and red meats can increase the risk of colon cancer. By making healthy food choices and focusing on a diet that is rich in colon-healthy foods, we can support the health of our gut and reduce the risk of colon cancer.

CHAPTER 8

Pancreatic Cancer Prevention – Foods to Support Pancreatic Health

Pancreatic cancer is one of the most aggressive and deadly forms of cancer. It is difficult to diagnose early and is often not detected until it has spread to other parts of the body. While there is no surefire way to prevent pancreatic cancer, recent research has shown that certain foods can help to support pancreatic health and reduce the risk of developing this devastating disease. In this chapter, we will explore the foods that can support pancreatic health and reduce the risk of pancreatic cancer.

Foods for Pancreatic Health

The pancreas is a crucial organ that plays a key role in digestion and the regulation of blood sugar levels. There are several foods that can support pancreatic health and help reduce the risk of pancreatic cancer. Fruits and vegetables, particularly those that are high in antioxidants, are excellent choices for pancreatic health. Antioxidants help to protect cells from damage caused by free radicals, which can contribute to the development of cancer. Berries, leafy greens, and cruciferous vegetables, such as broccoli and cauliflower, are particularly rich in antioxidants.

Omega-3 fatty acids are another nutrient that can support pancreatic health. Fatty fish, such as salmon and sardines, are excellent sources of omega-3 fatty acids. Additionally, plant-based sources of omega-3 fatty acids, such as flaxseeds, chia seeds, and walnuts, can also help to support pancreatic health.

Green tea is another food that has been shown to support pancreatic health. Green tea is rich in antioxidants and has been shown to have anti-cancer properties. Drinking green tea regularly may help to reduce the risk of pancreatic cancer.

Unhealthy Foods and Pancreatic Health

There are certain foods that can increase the risk of pancreatic cancer. A diet that is high in saturated and trans fats, for example, has been discovered to increase the risk of pancreatic cancer. Processed foods, such as chips, crackers, and baked goods, are often high in these unhealthy fats and should be avoided or limited in the diet.

Excessive alcohol consumption has also been linked to an increased risk of pancreatic cancer. It is important to limit alcohol consumption to no more than one drink per day for women and two drinks per day for men.

Conclusion

In conclusion, while there is no surefire way to prevent pancreatic cancer, there are various foods that can support the health of the pancreas and reduce the risk of developing this devastating disease. Fruits, vegetables, fatty fish, and green tea are all good choices for pancreatic health. In contrast, a diet that is high in unhealthy fats and excessive alcohol consumption can increase the risk of pancreatic cancer. By making healthy food choices and limiting our intake of unhealthy foods, we can support the health of our pancreas and reduce the risk of pancreatic cancer.

Part IV: Fighting Infection with Food

CHAPTER 9

Strengthening your immune system

The immune system is the body's defense against infections and diseases. It is a complex network of cells, tissues, and organs that work together to protect us from harmful pathogens like bacteria, viruses, and fungi. A strong immune system is essential for good health, as it can help to prevent infections and diseases from taking hold. In this chapter, we will explore the foods and lifestyle habits that can help to strengthen your immune system.

Foods to Boost Immune Function

One of the best ways to support immune function is to eat a diet that is rich in nutrient-dense foods. Foods that are high in vitamins A, C, and E, as well as zinc and selenium, are particularly beneficial for immune function. Some of the best foods for immune function include:

Citrus fruits like oranges, lemons, and grapefruits, which are high in vitamin C

Leafy greens like spinach, kale, and collard greens, are rich in vitamins A and E

Nuts and seeds like almonds, pumpkin seeds, and sunflower seeds, which are high in zinc and selenium

Garlic and ginger, have anti-inflammatory and immune-boosting properties

It is also important to include protein-rich foods in your diet, such as lean meats, poultry, fish, beans, and lentils. Protein is essential for the production of antibodies and other immune system components.

Lifestyle Habits for Strong Immune Function

In addition to eating a healthy diet, there are several lifestyle habits that can help to support immune function. These include:

Getting adequate sleep: Sleep is essential for immune function, as it allows the body to repair and regenerate.

Managing stress: Chronic stress can weaken the immune system, so it is important to find healthy ways to manage stress, such as meditation or yoga.

Exercising regularly: Regular exercise can help to boost immune function by improving blood circulation and reducing inflammation.

Avoiding smoking and excessive alcohol consumption: Both smoking and excessive alcohol consumption can weaken the immune system and increase the risk of infections and diseases.

Supplements for Immune Support

While it is best to get your nutrients from whole foods, some supplements can also help to support immune function. Some of the best supplements for immune support include:

Vitamin C: Vitamin C is a powerful antioxidant that can help to support immune function.

Vitamin D: Vitamin D is essential for immune function and can be difficult to get from food alone, particularly in the winter months.

Zinc: Zinc is important for immune function and can help to reduce the duration and severity of colds.

Conclusion

In conclusion, a strong immune system is essential for good health. By eating a diet that is rich in nutrient-dense foods, getting adequate sleep, managing stress, exercising regularly, and avoiding smoking and excessive alcohol consumption, we can help to support immune function. Additionally, some supplements, such as vitamin C, vitamin D, and zinc, can also help to boost immune function. By adopting these healthy habits, we can help to strengthen our immune systems and reduce the risk of infections and diseases.

Chapter 10

The American Meal Package: How It Contributes to Diabetes

Type 2 diabetes is a chronic condition that affects millions of people worldwide. It is characterized by high blood sugar levels, which can lead to a range of complications, including heart disease, nerve damage, and kidney failure. While there are many factors that contribute to the development of type 2 diabetes, diet is one of the most significant. In this chapter, we will explore the ways in which the American diet contributes to the development of type 2 diabetes.

The Standard American Meal (SAM)

The Standard American Meal is characterized by high levels of refined carbohydrates, processed foods, and added sugars. This diet is low in nutrient-dense foods like fruits, vegetables, and whole grains, which can contribute to nutrient deficiencies and poor overall health. The SAM is also high in saturated and trans fats, which can contribute to inflammation and insulin resistance.

Carbohydrates and Blood Sugar

Carbohydrates are an important source of energy for the body, but they can also contribute to high blood sugar levels. When we eat carbohydrates, they are broken down into glucose, which enters the bloodstream and raises blood sugar levels. This is particularly problematic for people with type 2 diabetes, as their bodies are less able to produce insulin, which is needed to transport glucose from the bloodstream into the cells.

Refined carbohydrates, such as white bread, pasta, and sugary drinks, are particularly problematic, as they are quickly broken down into glucose and can cause a rapid spike in blood sugar levels. This can put a strain on the body's insulin-producing cells and contribute to the development of insulin resistance, which is a precursor to type 2 diabetes.

Processed Foods and Added Sugars

Processed foods, such as packaged snacks and fast food meals, are often high in added sugars and unhealthy fats. These foods can contribute to inflammation and insulin resistance, which can increase the risk of type 2 diabetes. Added sugars, such as high-fructose corn syrup and table sugar, are particularly problematic, as they are quickly absorbed into the bloodstream and can cause a rapid spike in blood sugar levels.

Additionally, processed foods are often low in nutrient-dense foods like fruits, vegetables, and whole grains, which can contribute to nutrient deficiencies and poor overall health. Nutrient deficiencies, particularly in minerals like magnesium, have been linked to an increased risk of type 2 diabetes.

Healthy Eating for Diabetes Prevention and Management

To reduce the risk of type 2 diabetes and manage blood sugar levels, it is important to adopt a healthy diet that is rich in nutrient-dense foods and low in refined carbohydrates, processed foods, and added sugars.

Foods for the prevention and management of diabetes:

Non-starchy vegetables like broccoli, spinach, and kale, which are low in carbohydrates and high in fiber

Whole grains like quinoa, brown rice, and oatmeal, which are rich in fiber and other nutrients

Lean proteins like chicken, fish, and legumes, are important for maintaining muscle mass and reducing insulin resistance

Healthy fats like avocado, nuts, and olive oil, can help to reduce inflammation and improve insulin sensitivity

In addition to eating a healthy diet, it is also important to exercise regularly, manage stress, and maintain a healthy weight, as these factors can all contribute to diabetes prevention and management.

Conclusion

In conclusion, the American diet, characterized by high levels of refined carbohydrates, processed foods, and added sugars, can contribute to the development of type 2 diabetes. By adopting a healthy diet that is rich in nutrient-dense foods and low in refined carbohydrates, processed foods, and added sugars, we can reduce the risk of type 2 diabetes and manage blood sugar levels. It is also good to exercise regularly as it helps to manage stress.

CHAPTER 11

Reversing Diabetes: Foods to Regulate Blood Sugar

Diabetes is a chronic disease that affects millions of people worldwide. It is characterized by high blood sugar levels due to a lack of insulin or the body's inability to use insulin effectively. Poor dietary choices, lack of exercise, and genetics are all factors that contribute to the development of diabetes. Fortunately, research has shown that certain foods can help regulate blood sugar levels and even reverse the effects of diabetes.

In this chapter, we'll explore the foods that can help you manage and even reverse diabetes. We'll discuss the role of carbohydrates, protein, and fat in blood sugar regulation, as well as specific foods that can help balance blood sugar levels.

Carbohydrates are the primary source of energy for the body, but they can also cause blood sugar levels to spike. Therefore, it's important to choose carbohydrates that have a low glycemic index (GI). Foods with a low GI release glucose into the bloodstream slowly, helping to regulate blood sugar levels. Examples of low-GI foods include whole grains, legumes, and non-starchy vegetables.

Protein is also an essential nutrient for blood sugar regulation. It helps slow down the breakdown of carbohydrates and prevents blood sugar spikes.

It is also good to note that all proteins are not the same and equal. Animal protein, such as meat and dairy, has been shown to increase the risk of diabetes. On the other hand, plant-based proteins, such as beans, nuts, and seeds, have been shown to have a beneficial effect on blood sugar levels.

Fat is another important nutrient for blood sugar regulation. Healthy fats, such as those found in nuts, seeds, avocados, and fatty fish, have been shown to improve insulin sensitivity and lower the risk of diabetes. On the other hand, saturated and trans fats, found in processed foods and animal products, can increase insulin resistance and the risk of diabetes.

In addition to these nutrients, certain foods have been shown to have a specific impact on blood sugar levels. For example, cinnamon has been shown to improve insulin sensitivity and lower blood sugar levels in people with diabetes. Berries, especially blueberries, have been shown to improve insulin sensitivity and lower the risk of diabetes. Vinegar has also been discovered to improve insulin sensitivity and reduce blood sugar levels.

In conclusion, a healthy diet rich in whole grains, legumes, non-starchy vegetables, plant-based proteins, healthy fats, and specific blood sugar-regulating foods can help manage and even reverse the effects of diabetes. By making these dietary changes, you can take control of your blood sugar levels and improve your overall health.

CHAPTER 12

Understanding Hypertension: The Science Behind High Blood Pressure

High blood pressure, also known as hypertension, is a common condition that affects millions of people worldwide. It happens when the force of blood against the walls of the arteries is consistently too high. This can result in a variety of health challenges which include heart disease, stroke, and kidney failure. In this chapter, we'll explore the science behind high blood pressure, including its causes and risk factors, and how dietary choices can impact blood pressure levels.

Blood pressure is measured in two numbers: systolic pressure, which is the pressure when the heart beats, and diastolic pressure, which is the pressure when the heart is at rest between beats. A normal blood pressure reading is around 120/80 mmHg. Hypertension is defined as a blood pressure reading consistently higher than 140/90 mmHg.

There are several factors that can contribute to the development of hypertension, including genetics, age, and lifestyle factors such as diet and physical activity. Choices of diet are very important, as certain foods can contribute to high blood pressure.

Sodium or salt is a major agent in hypertension. Sodium causes the body to retain water and this increases the volume of blood and makes the arterial walls to be under pressure. Processed foods and restaurant meals are often high in sodium, making them a major contributor to hypertension.

Blood pressure can be regulated through the use of potassium. Potassium can help counteract the effects of sodium and help the body excrete excess sodium through the urine. Foods high in potassium include leafy greens, bananas, avocados, and sweet potatoes.

Other dietary factors that can impact blood pressure include alcohol consumption, caffeine intake, and sugar consumption. Alcohol and caffeine can both raise blood pressure, while excess sugar consumption can contribute to weight gain and obesity, which are risk factors for hypertension.

In addition to dietary changes, there are other lifestyle changes that can help manage hypertension, such as increasing physical activity, quitting smoking, and managing stress. Medications may also be necessary for some people with hypertension.

In conclusion, hypertension is a serious health condition that can lead to a variety of complications. However, by making dietary and lifestyle changes, it is possible to manage and even prevent hypertension.

By reducing sodium intake, increasing potassium intake, and making other healthy dietary choices, you can take control of your blood pressure and improve your overall health.

CHAPTER 13

Blood Pressure Control: Foods to Manage Hypertension

As discussed in the previous chapter, high blood pressure, or hypertension, is a serious health condition that can lead to a variety of complications. While lifestyle changes such as increasing physical activity, quitting smoking, and managing stress are important for managing hypertension, dietary choices can also play a significant role. In this chapter, we'll explore foods that can help manage hypertension and promote healthy blood pressure levels.

Reducing sodium intake is an important step in controlling blood pressure, as sodium is a major contributor to high blood pressure. Restricting or avoiding processed foods and restaurant dishes is key to reducing your sodium intake. These are often high in sodium. Instead, choose whole foods such as fruits, vegetables, whole grains, and lean protein.

Potassium is another key nutrient for blood pressure control. Potassium helps to counteract the effects of sodium and can help the body eliminate excess sodium through urine. The following food is high in potassium: bananas, avocados, leafy green, sweet potatoes, and tomatoes.

In addition to sodium and potassium, other nutrients that may play a role in blood pressure control include magnesium and calcium. Magnesium helps to relax blood vessels and can be found in foods such as nuts, seeds, legumes, and whole grains. Calcium promotes healthy blood vessel function and it can be found in dairy products, leafy greens, and fortified plant milk.

The DASH (Dietary Approaches to Stop Hypertension) diet is a dietary pattern that has been shown to be effective in managing hypertension. The DASH diet emphasizes fruits, vegetables, whole grains, lean proteins, and low-fat dairy products, while limiting processed foods, sodium, and added sugars.

In addition to dietary changes, other lifestyle factors can also help manage hypertension such as increasing physical activity, getting adequate sleep, managing stress etc. For some people, medications may also be necessary to manage blood pressure.

In summary, hypertension is a serious health condition that can be managed through a combination of lifestyle changes and dietary habits.

Reduce your sodium intake, increase your potassium intake, and make other healthy dietary choices. You can control your blood pressure and reduce your risk of complications such as heart disease, stroke, and kidney failure. See your doctor or licensed health care professional for personalized advice about managing high blood pressure with diet and lifestyle changes or consult a nutritionist.

CHAPTER 14

The Liver's Role in Overall Health: Foods to Prevent Liver Disease

The liver is a vital organ that plays a crucial role in overall health. It is responsible for filtering toxins from the body, producing bile to aid in digestion, and storing and releasing glucose for energy. However, a variety of factors such as poor diet, excessive alcohol consumption, and viral infections can cause damage to the liver and lead to liver disease. In this chapter, we'll explore foods that can help promote liver health and prevent liver disease.

One of the key nutrients for liver health is antioxidants. Antioxidants help to protect liver cells from damage caused by free radicals, which are unstable molecules that can cause cellular damage and inflammation. Foods that are high in antioxidants include berries, nuts, green tea, and dark chocolate.

Another important nutrient for liver health is fiber. Fiber helps to promote healthy digestion and can aid in the removal of toxins from the body. Foods that are rich in fiber include vegetables, whole grains, fruits, and legumes.

Sulfur-containing foods are also beneficial for liver health. Sulfur helps to promote the production of glutathione, a powerful antioxidant that plays a key role in liver function. Foods that are high in sulfur include garlic, onions, and cruciferous vegetables such as broccoli, Brussels sprouts, and cauliflower.

Additionally, certain vitamins and minerals are important for liver health. These include vitamins A, C, and E, as well as the minerals zinc and selenium. Vitamin A is found in foods such as carrots, sweet potatoes, and leafy greens. Vitamin C is found in citrus fruits, berries, and leafy greens. We can find Vitamin E in nuts, seeds, and vegetable oils. Zinc can be found in oysters, beef, and chicken, while selenium can be found in Brazil nuts, seafood, and poultry.

It's also important to reduce or stop taking certain foods that can contribute to liver damage. These include excessive alcohol consumption, high-fat and high-sugar foods, and processed foods. Instead, opt for whole foods such as fruits, vegetables, whole grains, lean proteins, and healthy fats.

In addition to dietary choices, there are other lifestyle factors that can help promote liver health. These include maintaining a healthy weight, avoiding smoking, and getting regular exercise.

In conclusion, the liver is a vital organ that plays a crucial role in overall health. By making healthy dietary choices and lifestyle changes, you can help promote liver health and prevent liver disease. Consult with a healthcare professional or registered dietitian for personalized advice on promoting liver health through diet and lifestyle changes.

CHAPTER 15

Managing Liver Disease: Foods to Support Liver Function

Liver disease is a serious condition that can have a significant impact on overall health. While there is no one-size-fits-all approach to managing liver disease, making healthy dietary choices can help support liver function and improve overall well-being. In this chapter, we'll explore foods that can be beneficial for individuals with liver disease.

Protein is an important nutrient for individuals with liver disease, as it helps to repair and regenerate liver tissue. However, it's important to choose the right type of protein. Opt for lean protein sources such as fish, poultry, beans, and lentils, rather than high-fat meats or processed meats, which can be harder for the liver to process.

Foods that are high in antioxidants are also beneficial for individuals with liver disease, as they can help to protect liver cells from further damage. Berries, nuts, green tea, and dark chocolate are all good sources of antioxidants.

In addition to antioxidants, certain vitamins, and minerals can be beneficial for individuals with liver disease. Vitamin E, for example, has been shown to have a protective effect on the liver. Foods that are high in vitamin E include nuts, seeds, and vegetable oils. Vitamin C is also important for liver health and can be found in citrus fruits, berries, and leafy greens. The mineral zinc is important for liver function and can be found in oysters, beef, and chicken.

Fiber is another important nutrient for individuals with liver disease. Fiber helps to promote healthy digestion and can aid in the removal of toxins from the body. Foods that are rich in fiber include vegetables, whole grains, fruits, and legumes.

It's also important to limit or avoid certain foods that can be hard on the liver. These include alcohol, high-fat and high-sugar foods, and processed foods. Additionally, individuals with liver disease may need to limit their intake of salt, as excessive sodium can contribute to fluid retention and swelling.

In addition to dietary choices, there are other lifestyle factors that can be helpful in managing liver disease. These include getting regular exercise, maintaining a healthy weight, and avoiding smoking.

It's important to work with a healthcare professional or registered dietitian to develop a personalized dietary plan for managing liver disease. Depending on the severity and type of liver disease, dietary recommendations may vary. In some cases, it may be necessary to limit certain nutrients or follow a specific dietary pattern.

In conclusion, making healthy dietary choices can help support liver function and improve overall well-being for individuals with liver disease. By choosing the right types of protein, incorporating antioxidant-rich foods, and focusing on fiber and important vitamins and minerals, individuals with liver disease can help support liver health. Consult with a healthcare professional or registered dietitian for personalized advice on managing liver disease through diet and lifestyle changes.

CHAPTER 16

Lymphoma Prevention and Treatment: Foods to Boost Immunity

Lymphoma is a type of cancer that affects the lymphatic system, which is part of the body's immune system. There are two main types of lymphoma:

1. Non-Hodgkin.

2. Hodgkin lymphoma.

There are several treatment options for lymphoma, but prevention through a healthy diet can greatly reduce your risk of developing the disease.

Foods rich in antioxidants, vitamins, and minerals can help boost the immune system and protect against cancer. Some of the best foods to eat for lymphoma prevention and treatment include:

Berries: Berries such as strawberries, blueberries, and raspberries are packed with antioxidants that can help protect cells from damage and reduce the risk of cancer.

Leafy greens: Dark and leafy greens such as spinach, collard greens etc are rich in minerals and vitamins that can help boost the immune system and protect against cancer.

Cruciferous vegetables: Vegetables such as broccoli, cauliflower, and Brussels sprouts contain compounds that can help prevent cancer and boost the immune system.

Citrus fruits: Citrus fruits such as oranges, lemons, and grapefruits are high in vitamin C, which is essential for a healthy immune system.

Garlic: Garlic contains compounds that can help reduce inflammation and protect against cancer.

Turmeric: Turmeric contains a compound called curcumin, which has been shown to have anti-cancer properties.

Green tea: Green tea contains antioxidants that can help protect against cancer and boost the immune system.

Whole grains: Whole grains such as brown rice, quinoa, and whole wheat bread are rich in fiber and nutrients that can help reduce the risk of cancer.

Legumes: Legumes such as beans, lentils, and chickpeas are rich in fiber and protein, and can help reduce the risk of cancer.

Nuts and seeds: Nuts and seeds such as almonds, walnuts, chia seeds, and flaxseeds are high in antioxidants and healthy fats that can help protect against cancer.

In addition to incorporating these foods into your diet, it's also important to limit processed foods, sugary drinks, and red meat, which have been linked to an increased risk of cancer.

It's important to note that while a healthy diet can help reduce the risk of developing lymphoma, it is not a guarantee of prevention or cure. It's always important to speak with a healthcare professional for personalized advice and treatment options.

CHAPTER 17

Leukemia Prevention and Treatment: Foods to Combat Cancer

Leukemia is a type of cancer that affects the blood and bone marrow, where the body produces blood cells. This disease can cause anemia, fatigue, infections, and easy bruising or bleeding. There are different types of leukemia, including acute lymphoblastic leukemia (ALL), acute myeloid leukemia (AML), chronic lymphocytic leukemia (CLL), and chronic myeloid leukemia (CML).

While leukemia can be treated with chemotherapy, radiation therapy, and stem cell transplant, there are also certain foods that can help prevent and combat the disease. In this chapter, we will explore the role of nutrition in leukemia prevention and treatment.

Fruits and vegetables

A diet rich in fruits and vegetables can help prevent leukemia by providing the body with antioxidants, vitamins, and minerals that support healthy immune function. Leafy greens, berries, citrus fruits, and cruciferous vegetables like broccoli and cauliflower are particularly beneficial. These foods contain compounds that have been shown to inhibit the growth of leukemia cells and promote their death.

Whole grains

Whole grains such as brown rice, quinoa, and whole-wheat bread are high in fiber and other nutrients that support overall health. These foods have also been found to reduce the risk of developing leukemia. One study showed that women who consumed more whole grains had a lower risk of developing leukemia than those who consumed less.

Lean protein

Lean protein sources like chicken, fish, and legumes are important for maintaining muscle mass and supporting immune function. These foods also contain amino acids that are essential for the production of white blood cells, which play a key role in fighting infections and diseases like leukemia.

Healthy fats

Healthy fats like those found in fatty fish, nuts, and seeds can help reduce inflammation in the body, which is important for preventing cancer. These foods also contain omega-3 fatty acids, which have been found to inhibit the growth of leukemia cells.

Green tea

Green tea contains catechins, which are compounds that have been found to have anti-cancer properties. Studies have shown that green tea can help prevent the development and progression of leukemia cells.

Turmeric

Turmeric is a spice that contains curcumin, a compound that has been found to have anti-inflammatory and anti-cancer properties. Curcumin has been shown to inhibit the growth of leukemia cells and induce their death.

Garlic

Garlic contains allicin, a compound that has been found to have anti-cancer properties. Studies have shown that garlic can help prevent the development of leukemia cells and reduce the risk of developing leukemia.

Berries

Berries contain anthocyanins, which are compounds that have been found to have anti-cancer properties. These compounds have been shown to inhibit the growth of leukemia cells and induce their death.

In conclusion, while a healthy diet cannot guarantee the prevention or treatment of leukemia, it can play an important role in supporting overall health and reducing the risk of developing cancer. By incorporating these foods into your diet, you can help support your immune system and reduce inflammation, which can ultimately contribute to a healthier body and a lower risk of leukemia.

CHAPTER 18

Multiple Myeloma Prevention and Treatment: Foods to Reduce Cancer Risk

Multiple myeloma is a cancer of the plasma cells, which are white blood cells that produce antibodies. While there is no cure for multiple myeloma, certain lifestyle choices, including diet, can play a role in prevention and treatment. In this chapter, we will discuss the foods that can reduce the risk of multiple myeloma and help those who are already living with this cancer.

Plant-based Foods: A plant-based diet is rich in phytochemicals and antioxidants, which can help prevent and fight cancer. Phytochemicals, found in fruits, vegetables, whole grains, and legumes, have been shown to have anti-cancer properties. Antioxidants, found in brightly colored fruits and vegetables, help to reduce inflammation and oxidative stress, which are factors that can contribute to cancer development. Include a variety of plant-based foods in your diet to reap the benefits of these nutrients.

Omega-3 Fatty Acids: Omega-3 fatty acids are a type of healthy fat that are found in fatty fish, such as salmon and sardines, as well as in flaxseed, chia seeds, and walnuts. Studies have shown that omega-3 fatty acids have anti-inflammatory properties that may reduce the risk of multiple myeloma. Incorporate these foods into your diet to reap the benefits of omega-3 fatty acids.

Turmeric: Turmeric is a spice that is commonly used in Indian cuisine and has been shown to have anti-cancer properties. Curcumin, the active compound in turmeric, has been found to inhibit the growth and spread of cancer cells in multiple myeloma. Consider adding turmeric to your meals or taking a turmeric supplement to reap the benefits of this powerful spice.

Green Tea: Green tea is a rich source of polyphenols, which are antioxidants that can help prevent cancer. Studies have shown that green tea may reduce the risk of multiple myeloma by inhibiting the growth and spread of cancer cells. Consider swapping out your daily cup of coffee for green tea to reap the benefits of this cancer-fighting beverage.

Cruciferous Vegetables: Cruciferous vegetables, such as broccoli, cauliflower, and kale, are rich in sulfur-containing compounds called glucosinolates. These compounds have been shown to have anti-cancer properties and may reduce the risk of multiple myeloma. Include these vegetables in your diet to benefit from their cancer-fighting properties.

Probiotics: Probiotics are beneficial bacteria that are found in fermented foods, such as yogurt, kefir, and sauerkraut. These bacteria have been shown to support gut health and boost the immune system, which can help prevent cancer. Consider incorporating probiotic-rich foods into your diet to reap the benefits of these beneficial bacteria.

In addition to these specific foods, it is important to maintain an overall healthy and balanced diet to reduce the risk of multiple myeloma. This includes limiting processed and high-fat foods, choosing lean protein sources, and staying hydrated by drinking plenty of water. By making these dietary changes, individuals can reduce their risk of multiple myeloma and improve their overall health.

CHAPTER 19

Making It Stick: Tips for Incorporating Disease-Fighting Foods into Your Diet

Now that you've learned about the various foods that can prevent and reverse diseases, it's time to incorporate them into your diet. However, making changes to your diet can be challenging, especially if you are used to eating a certain way. In this chapter, we will explore some tips and strategies that can help you make these changes stick.

Set realistic goals: Start small and work your way up. Instead of trying to change your entire diet at once, set smaller, more manageable goals, such as incorporating one new fruit or vegetable into your meals each week.

Plan your meals: Plan your meals in advance to ensure that you have healthy options on hand. This can help you avoid reaching for less healthy options when you're hungry and pressed for time.

Keep healthy snacks on hand: Stock up on healthy snacks, such as nuts, seeds, and fresh fruit, to help you avoid reaching for unhealthy snacks when you're hungry.

Get creative in the kitchen: Experiment with different recipes and cooking methods to make your meals more interesting and flavorful.

Seek support: Join a support group or enlist the help of family and friends to help you stay motivated and accountable.

Be patient: Remember that change takes time and that slip-ups are a normal part of the process. Don't get discouraged if you have setbacks, and keep working towards your goals.

Stay informed: Continue to educate yourself on the benefits of healthy eating, and keep up-to-date on the latest research in the field.

By incorporating these strategies into your daily routine, you can increase your chances of success and make healthy eating a lifelong habit. Remember that the foods you choose to eat can have a powerful impact on your health, so make your choices wisely.

CHAPTER 20

The Future of Food and Disease Prevention: A Look Ahead

As our understanding of the relationship between food and disease continues to grow, it's becoming increasingly clear that the food we eat can have a profound impact on our health. But what does the future hold in terms of using food to prevent and treat disease? In this chapter, we'll explore some of the exciting research and innovations that are shaping the future of food and disease prevention.

Precision Nutrition

One of the most exciting developments in the field of nutrition is the idea of precision nutrition. Precision nutrition takes into account an individual's unique genetic makeup, lifestyle, and health status to create personalized dietary recommendations. This approach recognizes that there is no generalized approach to nutrition and that the foods that are beneficial for one person may not be as beneficial for another.

In recent years, advances in technology have made precision nutrition more accessible than ever before. For example, at-home genetic testing kits can provide individuals with information about their genetic predisposition to certain diseases, as well as insights into how their bodies metabolize different nutrients.

This information can be used to create personalized nutrition plans that are tailored to an individual's unique needs.

Functional Foods

Another area of research that is shaping the future of food and disease prevention is the development of functional foods. Functional foods are foods that have been fortified with specific nutrients or compounds that are known to have health benefits beyond basic nutrition.

For example, some foods may be fortified with probiotics, which are beneficial bacteria that live in the gut and have been shown to support digestive health and boost the immune system. Other foods may be fortified with antioxidants, which help to protect cells from damage caused by free radicals and may help to reduce the risk of chronic diseases such as cancer and heart disease.

The development of functional foods is still in its early stages, but there is a great deal of interest in this area among researchers and food manufacturers alike. As more is learned about the specific compounds that can have a positive impact on health, we can expect to see more foods being fortified with these compounds.

Plant-Based Proteins

As concerns about the environmental impact of animal agriculture continue to grow, there is increasing interest in plant-based proteins as a more sustainable and ethical source of protein. Plant-based proteins such as soy, peas, and quinoa are already widely available, but there is a growing push to develop even more plant-based protein sources.

One of the most exciting developments in this area is the development of lab-grown meat. Lab-grown meat is created by growing animal cells in a lab, rather than raising and slaughtering animals. While this technology is still in its early stages, it has the potential to revolutionize the meat industry and make meat production much more sustainable.

Conclusion

As our understanding of the relationship between food and disease continues to grow, there is no doubt that the future of food and disease prevention is a bright one. From precision nutrition to functional foods to plant-based proteins, there is a wide range of exciting innovations and developments on the horizon that have the potential to transform the way we think about food and health. By staying up-to-date with the latest research and developments in this field, we can all take steps to improve our health and prevent disease.